MA

A manual

healtl

World Hea

C

12/5/98
M

WHO Library Cataloguing in Publication Data
Malaria: a manual for community health workers.

    1.Malaria   2.Community health aides   3.Manuals

    ISBN 92 4 154491 0   (NLM Classification: WC 750)

The World Health Organization welcomes requests for permission to reproduce or translate its publications, in part or in full. Applications and enquiries should be addressed to the Office of Publications, World Health Organization, Geneva, Switzerland, which will be glad to provide the latest information on any changes made to the text, plans for new editions, and reprints and translations already available.

The designations employed and the presentation of the material in this publication do not imply the expression of any opinion whatsoever on the part of the Secretariat of the World Health Organization concerning the legal status of any country, territory, city or area or of its authorities, or concerning the delimitation of its frontiers or boundaries.

The mention of specific companies or of specific manufacturers' products does not imply that they are endorsed or recommended by the World Health Organization in preference to others of a similar nature that are not mentioned. Errors and omissions excepted, the names of proprietary products are distinguished by initial capital letters.

TYPESET IN HONG KONG
PRINTED IN ENGLAND

95/10714—Best-set/Clays—8000

As a community health worker you can help your village, your family, and yourself to control malaria:

- Prompt treatment of malaria saves lives

- Prompt treatment of malaria reduces the duration of disease and its harmful effects on the human body

- Preventive measures in the community reduce the risk of people getting malaria

Contents

Preface

This manual has been prepared by Dr R. L. Kouznetsov, Malaria Control, in collaboration with Dr P. F. Beales, Chief, Training, Division of Control of Tropical Diseases, World Health Organization, for the training of community health workers in malaria control. It may also be used by community health workers to support their day-to-day work.

The manual contains the basic information and guidance required for the recognition of malaria, its treatment, and identification of cases to be referred; recording and reporting; promotion of community awareness about malaria; and promotion of relevant and feasible preventive activities.

It is emphasized that this manual should serve as a basis for local adaptation, since the epidemiological, social, and economic conditions—as well as health care delivery systems and approaches to malaria treatment and control—vary considerably from country to country and even within each country. Enquiries regarding adaptation are welcomed, and should be addressed in the first instance to the Office of Publications, World Health Organization, 1211 Geneva 27, Switzerland. The text is available from WHO on computer diskette to make adaptation easier.

Staff of national malaria control programmes should note the following:

- It is normally the responsibility of national malaria control programmes to define the first-line treatment for uncomplicated malaria to be used by community health workers. This manual has been written with chloroquine as the first-line treatment. Where chloroquine is not the first-line treatment, the manual must be modified accordingly.
- On page 27 the community health worker is advised to ask his or her supervisor about whether malaria is common in the area. Thus, for optimal use of this manual, community health worker supervisors must be informed as to whether their area is classed as one of high or low malaria risk. In

countries where malaria is highly endemic, it is safe to assume that malaria is common in the community health worker's area.

Comments and suggestions arising from the practical use of this manual would be greatly appreciated, and should be addressed to Training, Division of Control of Tropical Diseases, World Health Organization, 1211 Geneva 27, Switzerland.

Acknowledgements

The Malaria Division, Ministry of Health and Medical Services, Solomon Islands, allowed extensive use of their national guidelines for primary health workers. The World Health Organization gratefully acknowledges the role of this valuable partnership in the preparation of this manual. The authors also wish to thank the staff of the Malaria Control and Training units of WHO's Division of Control of Tropical Diseases, for their constructive criticism and encouragement during the preparation phase; particular thanks are owed to Dr A. Shapira for his valuable contributions and to the WHO Regional Offices.

Part 1
Introduction

What you can do about malaria

Malaria is one of the most serious diseases to affect people in developing countries with tropical and subtropical climates. It is particularly dangerous for young children and for pregnant women and their unborn children, although others may be seriously affected in some circumstances.

Malaria is a curable and preventable disease, but it still kills many people. The main reasons for this unsatisfactory situation are:

- Some people do not come for treatment until they are very ill because:
    — they do not realize they might have malaria (people often think they have a cold, influenza or other common infection);
    — they do not realize that malaria is very dangerous; or
    — they live far away from health care facilities.
- People living far from health services will often go to local medicine vendors (sellers) for advice, which is not always appropriate, or to buy medicines, which are not always effective.
- Many people do not know what causes malaria or how it is spread, so they are not able to protect themselves from the disease.

As a community health worker you can improve the situation by performing the following activities:

- Encourage people to seek treatment *immediately* if they have fever. This is especially important in young children and pregnant women, who should receive treatment against malaria within 24 hours of becoming ill.
- Recognize and treat malaria to prevent severe illness and death.
- Explain how to take treatment correctly, so that people can avoid repeated attacks of malaria.
- Advise patients who do not improve within 48 hours after starting treatment, or whose condition is serious, to go

immediately to the nearest hospital or clinic capable of making a definite diagnosis and managing severe disease.

- Advise individuals and families on how to protect themselves from mosquito bites.
- Motivate the community to carry out mosquito control measures in order to reduce the number of malaria cases.

All of these activities are explained in this manual.

Remember:

Prompt treatment of malaria saves lives

Prompt treatment of malaria reduces the duration of disease and its harmful effects on the human body

Preventive measures in the community reduce the risk of people getting malaria

---

Medicines and equipment you will need

You should have the following items in your medical kit:

- **Antimalarial drug(s)***

- **Paracetamol or acetylsalicylic acid (aspirin)**

- **Treatment schedule**

- **Pencils and paper**

- **A day-book and a monthly report form**

- **Malaria health education materials**

- **A copy of this book**

It is your responsibility to have enough drugs at all times because the community will come to rely on you for treatment and advice. Always use up older medicines before you start using any new supplies.

Drugs should be kept indoors away from sunlight and heat, preferably in a locked box or cupboard, out of children's reach. Remember, **it is very dangerous to swallow large quantities of antimalaria drugs** at the same time.

---

* Your government's Ministry of Health should specify which antimalarial drug(s) may be used by community health workers and how they should be given—ask your supervisor.

Part 2
General information about malaria and its prevention

What are the effects of malaria?

Malaria is a disease that is caused by the presence of very small organisms (malaria parasites) in the blood. Malaria parasites are so small that they can only be seen under a microscope. They feed on the blood cells, multiply inside them and destroy them.

Later (pages 23–28) you will learn how to recognize malaria in a sick person. It is often difficult to tell whether a sickness is caused by malaria or some other disease, because the features may be similar. Therefore, if the patient's condition has not improved within 2 days after the start of an adequate malaria treatment, he or she needs urgent care in the nearest clinic or hospital (see page 37).

Malaria is especially dangerous in pregnant women and, in particular, young children (under 5 years old). If a pregnant woman or young child gets malaria, severe illness may rapidly develop and may even result in death. Such patients need special care in addition to standard malaria treatment (see "Special groups, special care" (page 39)).

In areas where malaria is very common, people may get the disease several times during their lives. This gives them some resistance to the disease, so the attacks of malaria often become less severe as they get older.

However, adults who come from areas where malaria is not common can become very ill with malaria, just like children.

> **Malaria is especially dangerous for young children and pregnant women**

How do people get malaria?

The malaria parasites enter and leave the body through
mosquito bites (see Fig. 1).

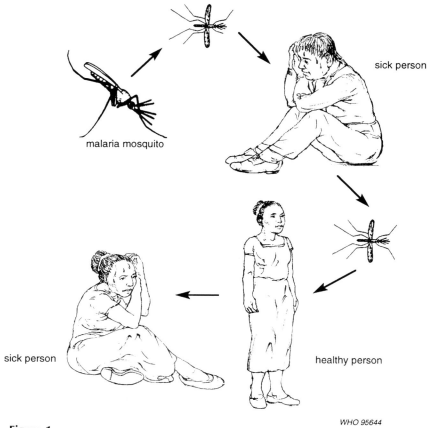

malaria mosquito

sick person

healthy person

sick person

WHO 95644

Figure 1

- When a mosquito bites a person it sucks up blood. If the
  person has malaria, some of the parasites in the blood will be
  sucked into the mosquito.
- The malaria parasites multiply and develop in the mosquito.
  After 10–14 days they are mature and ready to be passed on
  to someone else.

• If the mosquito now bites a healthy person, the malaria parasites will enter the body of the healthy person. This person will then become ill.

Mosquitos may bite people with malaria, and then pass it on to many other people in the village

How do malaria mosquitos live?

There are many different kinds of mosquitos, but only *malaria mosquitos* can pass on malaria parasites. All malaria mosquitos have white and black spots on their wings (but a mosquito with white and black spots is not necessarily a malaria mosquito).

Only *female* mosquitos bite people. Male mosquitos do not suck up blood and cannot pass on malaria parasites. Female mosquitos need blood to produce eggs. The eggs are very small: you can hardly see them. They are laid on *stagnant or slow-flowing water*. Usually the mosquitos that bite you are breeding in collections of water within 2 kilometres (about 1.25 miles) of the place where you live.

Two or three days after the eggs are laid on the water, a mosquito *larva* will come out of each egg. The larva feeds on very small animals and plants in the water, and grows until it becomes a *pupa*. The pupa remains in the water, but does not feed. After a few days the *adult* mosquito will come out of the pupa and fly away. If it is a female mosquito, it may bite people and feed on their blood. After feeding, the mosquito usually rests on a nearby surface before it flies away. Then it will lay eggs and everything starts all over again. In tropical countries it takes 7–14 days for a mosquito to grow from an egg to an adult mosquito (see Fig. 2).

A mosquito egg, larva or pupa does not have malaria parasites inside it. Adult mosquitos may have malaria parasites in their bodies, but only if they have bitten someone who has malaria.

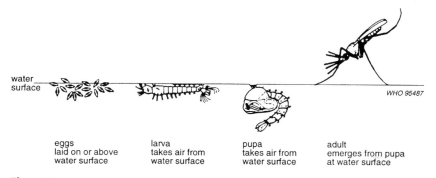

water surface

WHO 95487

eggs
laid on or above
water surface

larva
takes air from
water surface

pupa
takes air from
water surface

adult
emerges from pupa
at water surface

Figure 2

How can you prevent malaria?

There are three main ways to prevent malaria:

1. **Prevent mosquitos from biting people:**
   — sleep under mosquito nets (ordinary or insecticide-treated);
   — screen all windows and doors in the house, or at least in rooms where people sleep;
   — apply mosquito repellents to the skin;
   — burn mosquito coils.

2. **Control mosquito breeding:**
   — eliminate places where mosquitos can lay eggs;
   — reclaim land by filling and draining;
   — introduce special fish that eat mosquito larvae;
   — put special insecticides in the water to kill mosquito larvae.

3. **Kill adult mosquitos:**
   — spray rooms with insecticides before going to bed;
   — participate in activities carried out by the health services, such as spraying the inside walls of houses with insecticides that kill mosquitos.

Some of the activities mentioned under "Control mosquito breeding" are complex and expensive. House spraying campaigns are also expensive. These methods need planning and supervision by specialized staff.

The measures described in the following pages can be applied by individuals and communities with your advice and guidance. Discuss with your supervisor the possibility of applying some of these measures to your area.

If you apply these measures correctly, you will reduce the risk of malaria for everyone in your village. You will probably not be able to get rid of malaria from your village completely (it is usually impossible to eliminate all breeding places), but you can greatly reduce the number of people who get malaria.

How to prevent mosquito bites

Mosquito nets

A mosquito net (Fig. 3) is a very good way to protect people from getting malaria. Mosquito nets do not kill mosquitos, but while you are underneath them the mosquitos cannot bite you.

Malaria mosquitos usually bite from sunset to sunrise. Therefore mosquito nets are especially good for protecting young children who are already asleep by sunset. Nets are also good for protecting older children and adults because some mosquitos bite during the night.

Malaria is particularly dangerous for young children and pregnant women (see pages 39–40). It is therefore very important that they use mosquito nets. Young children and pregnant women should go to sleep early (under mosquito nets) to avoid mosquito bites during the evening.

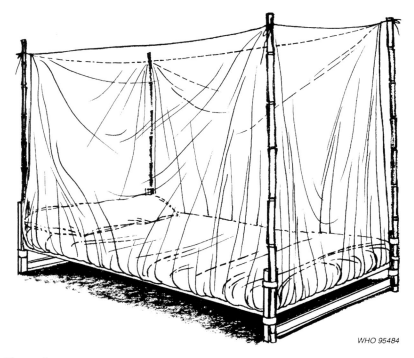

WHO 95484

Figure 3

Mosquito nets will not prevent malaria unless they are used correctly:

- Torn sections must be repaired.
- Mosquito nets should be hung up properly to cover the sleeping area and should be low enough to allow netting to be tucked in under the mattress or mat where the person sleeps.
- Mosquitos that are trapped inside the net should be killed with insecticide spray or by hand.

Mosquito nets provide much better protection if they are treated with a special insecticide. This insecticide is not harmful to people if used correctly, but it kills mosquitos and keeps them away from the house. Treated nets also kill bed bugs and other insects. Insecticides are useful, but they are dangerous if used incorrectly. You must receive special training before you can advise people on how to treat nets with insecticides.

Screening

A single mosquito net provides protection only for those sleeping under it, but screening the house will protect the whole family (Fig. 4).

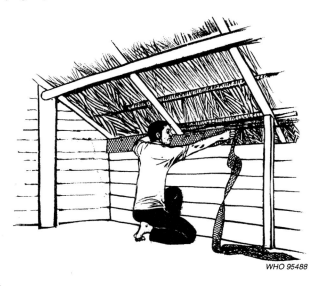

WHO 95488

Figure 4

15

Effective screening is possible only in houses that are well constructed and maintained. Various materials (usually metal or plastic) can be used for screening. Frequent inspection is necessary to detect damage to the screens and to make early repairs.

Another way of keeping out mosquitos is to use curtains made from netting or similar materials. These curtains must be treated regularly with a special insecticide and they must be hung up in such a way that they cover all openings to the house.

Repellents

Repellents are chemicals that you apply to the skin to keep mosquitos away (Fig. 5). They are sold in pharmacies and some other shops. Repellents prevent mosquitos from landing on your body.

Repellents are very useful early in the evening (when people are not under mosquito nets or inside screened houses). They are usually active for 5–8 hours, then they have to be applied again.

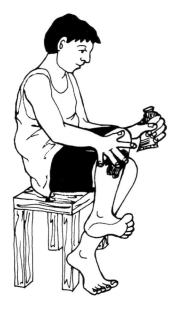

Figure 5

Mosquito coils

When mosquito coils burn, their smoke keeps mosquitos away.
If mosquitos fly through the smoke, they may even be killed.
The coils are not very expensive and (like the repellents) are
especially useful early in the evening when people sit outdoors
(Fig. 6).

How to control mosquito breeding

Malaria mosquitos may breed in:

— freshwater or brackish (slightly salty) water, especially if it
   is stagnant or slow-flowing;
— open streams with very slow-flowing water along their banks;
— pools of water left on the riverbed after the rains have
   ended, or as a result of poor water management;

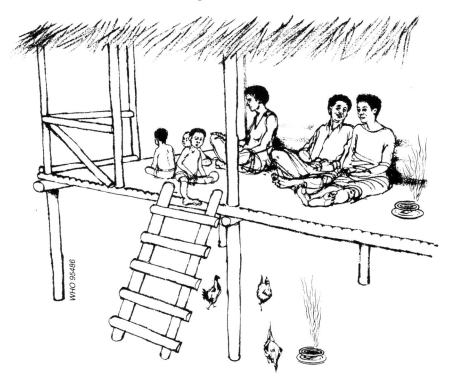

WHO 95486

Figure 6

— swamps, rice fields, and reservoirs;
— small ponds, pools, borrow-pits, canals, and ditches with stagnant water, in and around villages;
— animal hoof-prints filled with water;
— cisterns (water tanks) for storage of water; and
— anything that may collect water—plant pots, old car tyres, etc.

Remember—the mosquitos that bite you usually breed within 2 kilometres (1.25 miles) of where you live.

Individuals and communities can reduce mosquito breeding by the following activities:

• Use sand to fill in pools, ponds, borrow-pits, and hoof-prints in and around the village (Fig. 7).
• Remove discarded containers that might collect water.
• Cover cisterns (water tanks) with mosquito nets or lids.
• Clear away vegetation and other matter from the banks of streams—this will speed up the flow of water.
• Pools of water may be caused by leaking taps, spillage of water around stand-pipes and wells, or poor drains. These

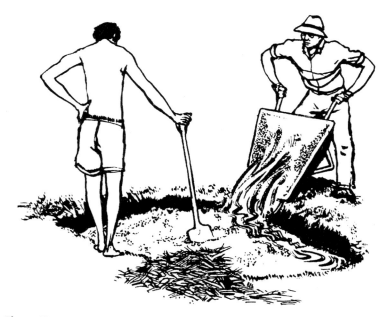

Figure 7

pools can be eliminated by repairs or improvements to the water supply or drainage system.

Elimination of mosquito breeding in large expanses of water (or in areas where small pools of water are abundant after the rains) usually requires major engineering works.

Whenever you have a problem, ask your supervisor for advice; if he or she does not know the answer immediately, specialists in malaria and environmental health can be contacted for advice and help.

Remember, you can only control malaria in your village if everybody works together to carry out these measures. The village needs to be organized so that everybody is involved in mosquito control. Read "How to organize your village" (Annex 2 on page 45).

Part 3
Recognition and treatment of malaria

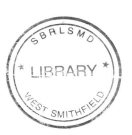

Take enough time to pay proper attention to what the patient has to say and to examine the patient in order to recognize disease correctly

Provide appropriate treatment without delay

Do not try to treat a patient who requires medical care that is beyond your skills and competence—always refer such patients for expert consultation and treatment

Clinical features of malaria

The clinical features of malaria vary from very mild to very severe, depending on several factors. For example, in areas where malaria is very common, adults with the disease might have just a slight increase in body temperature. However, pregnant women and, in particular, young children often have a severe illness with many symptoms and signs, and they may even die.

The most important feature of malaria is fever (or a history of fever within the last 2–3 days). The fever may be either continuous or irregular at the start of the illness, but soon it may become regular, with attacks every 2–3 days.

Each attack may last several hours and often begins with shivering (body shaking); then there is a period of fever, and finally there is profuse sweating. During an attack the patient often complains of headache and pains in the back, joints, and all over the body. There may also be loss of appetite, vomiting, and diarrhoea.

The patient may feel better the next day, but has another attack the day after that, and so on. If untreated (or inadequately treated), malaria may cause several weeks or months of poor health because of repeated attacks of fever, anaemia (see page 26), and general weakness.

Some patients (usually young children) rapidly become very ill and may die within a few days (see "Danger signs of severe malaria", page 24).

How to recognize malaria

You can recognize malaria by *asking* and *looking* (whether you are in a clinic, a health centre, or the patient's home):

1. *Ask* questions and listen to what the patient has to say (if the patient is a young child, listen to the parent or guardian).
2. *Look*—examine the patient for features of malaria.

Start by asking why the patient (or parent) is seeking your help. Malaria is a possibility if one of the complaints is FEVER. If the patient (or parent) does not mention fever, ask whether there has been a fever at any time during the past 2–3 days. In some places, it is better to ask whether the patient has felt hot or cold, or whether the child's body has felt hot to touch.

Measure the temperature with a thermometer. If the temperature is more than 37.5 °C, the patient has a fever. (If you do not have a thermometer with you, feel the forehead with the back of your hand. If the forehead feels hot, the patient probably has a fever.)

If there is no fever, and no history of fever during the past 2–3 days, the patient does *not* have malaria.

Patients who have had fever during the last 2–3 days *may* have malaria.

If the patient has had fever during the past 2–3 days, first *ask* about and then *look* for danger signs.

Danger signs of severe malaria

The danger signs of malaria are:

— changes in behaviour (convulsions; unconsciousness; sleepiness; confusion; inability to walk, sit, speak, or recognize relatives);

— repeated vomiting; inability to retain oral medication; inability to eat or to drink;
— passage of small quantities of urine or no urine, or passage of dark urine;
— severe diarrhoea;
— unexplained heavy bleeding from nose, gums, or other sites;
— high fever (above 39 °C);
— severe dehydration (loose skin and sunken eyes);
— anaemia (see page 26);
— yellow whites of eyes.

If you see any of these features you should think about malaria and act immediately (see page 38).

How to recognize the danger signs

Ask:

- Is the patient unable to drink?
- Has the patient had convulsions (fits)?
- Does the patient vomit repeatedly?
- How much urine does the patient pass?—Very little? None at all? Is it dark?

Look:

- Is the patient abnormally sleepy, difficult to wake, or confused?
- Does the patient have anaemia (see box below)?
- Does the patient have severe dehydration? (Look for sudden weight loss, loose skin, sunken eyes, dry mouth. Dehydration is always important to recognize—for more details, refer to the notes from your diarrhoea course or your general course.)
- Is the patient unable to stand or sit?

If the answer to any of these questions is yes, the patient has severe febrile disease—probably severe malaria. The patient's life is in danger. Urgent treatment is needed at a clinic or hospital to save the patient's life.

Give the first dose of antimalaria treatment. Then refer the patient to the nearest clinic or hospital. Write a referral note to go with the patient; include details of what you have observed and what treatment you have given and when.

If you think a person has severe malaria, you must act immediately—read "Severe malaria" (page 38) for details of what to do.

Anaemia

Anaemia means "not enough haemoglobin in the blood". Haemoglobin is the red substance in the blood cells which carries oxygen. Malaria parasites destroy the blood cells, and so malaria may cause anaemia. Anaemia may also have other causes (for example, not enough iron in the food).

You can recognize anaemia by looking at the patient's hands: the palms of a patient with anaemia do not have the redness of a healthy person's palms.

If you are not sure, look at the red of the eye by carefully pulling down the lower eyelid with clean fingers. Look also in the mouth. If the red colour of the eye or mouth is paler than in a healthy person, the patient has anaemia.

Anaemia is less noticeable than other danger signs, but it is dangerous. Start treatment against malaria and refer the patient to a hospital or clinic.

If there are no danger signs

If the patient has had a fever during the past 2–3 days, he or she may have malaria.

Ask your supervisor whether malaria is present in your area.

How often does it occur?

Where is it most common?

Does it occur at certain times of year?

In many areas malaria occurs during and after the rainy season; in other areas (particularly areas that are hot and humid, and full of places where mosquitos breed) malaria is common all year round.

If you know how common malaria is in your area, this will help you assess the risk of exposure and the chances that your patient may have the disease.

If you work in an area where malaria is abundant

A child less than 5 years old or a pregnant woman (especially if she is pregnant for the first time) who has had fever at any time during the past 2–3 days should be treated for malaria immediately, because malaria can rapidly become dangerous in young children and pregnant women. You should refer all pregnant women who are suspected to have malaria to the nearest clinic or hospital. At the same time look for signs and symptoms of other diseases and treat them accordingly.

If the patient is more than 5 years old, look for other causes of fever as described below. If you cannot find another cause for the fever, the patient probably has malaria.

If you work in an area where malaria is not common

First, find out whether the patient has a fever or has had a fever within the past 2–3 days (see page 24).

If the patient does not have fever when examined by you and does not have a history of fever within the past 2–3 days, he or she does *not* have malaria.

A patient with fever (or a recent history of fever) may or may not have malaria:

- If the patient has a runny nose, measles, an abscess, earache, or signs and symptoms of any other well known causes of fever, he or she probably does not have malaria. (Measles is a disease of children. Its features are red eyes, sore mouth, and rash. You learn to recognize it by observing sick children together with someone who is very experienced. An abscess is a tender, hot swelling somewhere on the body.)
- If the patient does not have a runny nose, measles, abscess, etc., but does have fever or a recent history of fever, the patient may have malaria, especially if he or she is seen during the malaria season.

- **Early diagnosis and adequate treatment are essential in young children and pregnant women, otherwise they may die**

- **Do not try to manage a patient who requires medical care that is beyond your skills and competence**

- **Do not be afraid to refer sick patients for expert consultation and treatment—know and respect your own limitations**

Pneumonia

Young children with malaria often have pneumonia at the same time. A child probably has pneumonia if he or she:

— is 2–12 months of age and breathes 50 times per minute or more;
— is between 12 months and 5 years of age and breathes 40 times per minute or more.

If you have learned how to manage pneumonia, proceed accordingly (treat cases of simple pneumonia; refer cases of severe pneumonia). If you have not learned how to manage pneumonia, refer any child with signs of pneumonia but, if the child has had fever during the past 2–3 days, start treatment for malaria—give the first dose of standard malaria treatment and then refer to a clinic or hospital.

How to give standard malaria treatment

Before you give treatment, check whether the patient has already been treated for malaria in the past 14 days. If so, the patient has a *treatment failure*—read page 37 before you give any further treatment.

If the patient has not received treatment for malaria in the past 14 days, you must give standard malaria treatment. Go through the following steps in the order shown:

1. Fill in the necessary forms (see "Recording and reporting", page 41).
2. Supervise treatment (see below, "How to supervise treatment").
3. If the patient lives far away, you may need to make special arrangements (see "If supervision is impossible", page 34).

How to supervise treatment

Chloroquine is the standard treatment for malaria in most countries (check with your supervisor). The number of tablets you need to give depends on the weight of the patient. Small children weigh less than adults and therefore they need less medicine than adults.

If you cannot weigh your patient, you can work out how many tablets to give according to the patient's age. Tables 1, 2, and 3 show you how to do this. If your tablets contain 100 mg chloroquine per tablet, use Table 1. If they contain 150 mg per tablet, use Table 2. If you are using chloroquine syrup (50 mg per 5 ml) to treat a young child, use Table 3.

Always follow the correct treatment schedules. If you do not give enough medicine, the patient will not be cured of malaria. If you give too much, this can also be harmful to health.

Table 1
How many chloroquine tablets you should give if each tablet contains chloroquine 100 mg[a]

Day	Age (years)				
	under 1	1 – 3	4 – 6	7 –11	over 11
Day 1	1	1½	2	3½	6
Day 2	1	1½	2	3½	6
Day 3	½	½	1	1½	2½

WHO 95639

[a] For example, if your patient is aged between 7 and 11 years, you should give 3½ tablets on day 1, 3½ tablets on day 2, and 1½ tablets on day 3.

Table 2
How many chloroquine tablets you should give if each tablet contains chloroquine 150 mg[a]

Day	Age (years)				
	under 1	1 – 3	4 – 6	7 –11	over 11
Day 1	½	1	1½	2½	4
Day 2	½	1	1½	2½	4
Day 3	½	½	½	1	2

WHO 95640

[a] For example, if your patient is aged between 7 and 11 years, you should give 2½ tablets on day 1, 2½ tablets on day 2, and 1 tablet on day 3.

Table 3
How many 5-ml spoonfuls you should give if you are using chloroquine syrup 50 mg per 5 ml[a,b]

Day	Age (years)	
	under 1	1 – 3
Day 1	5 ml 2.5 ml TOTAL = 7.5 ml	5 ml 5 ml 5 ml TOTAL = 15 ml
Day 2	5 ml 2.5 ml TOTAL = 7.5 ml	5 ml 5 ml 5 ml TOTAL = 15 ml
Day 3	5 ml TOTAL = 5 ml	5 ml TOTAL = 5 ml

WHO 95641

a For example, if your patient is less than 1 year old, you should give 1 1/2 spoonfuls on day 1, 1 1/2 spoonfuls on day 2, and 1 spoonful on day 3.

b Always use special 5-ml spoons for giving medicine, otherwise the amount you give will not be accurate.

Pregnant women with malaria must take the full dose of chloroquine like all malaria patients. Chloroquine will not harm the unborn child, but malaria will if it is not treated properly.

If possible, supervise treatment. This means that you watch the patient swallow the chloroquine tablets on *all 3 days* of treatment. This is to make sure the patient takes the tablets properly, and also to make sure that he or she does not vomit.

Always make sure the patient drinks enough water to make the tablets go down. Tablets should not be taken on an empty stomach, because this is likely to cause vomiting and abdominal pain, especially in children.

Crying children will not swallow medicine—they will spit it out! Wait for a few minutes to let them calm down before you give the medicine.

If the patient vomits within 30 minutes after taking the medicine, let the person rest a little and try to give the medicine once again. Crush the tablets and mix the powder with some sugar and water, particularly if the patient is a child.

If the patient vomits again and again, refer to a clinic or hospital.

> **If there is no improvement within 48 hours after swallowing the first dose of the treatment, the patient should be taken to the nearest clinic or hospital**

If your patient has a high fever, you can give paracetamol. The number of tablets you should give depends on the amount of paracetamol in each tablet (100 mg or 500 mg) and the age of the patient (see Tables 4 and 5). Paracetamol will reduce the temperature in about 1 hour.

If paracetamol is not available, you can give acetylsalicylic acid (aspirin) instead. The dose (in milligrams) is the same as for paracetamol. However, the actual number of tablets you should give depends on how many milligrams there are in each tablet. Work out with your supervisor how many tablets you should give for each age group.

Table 4
How many paracetamol tablets you should give if each tablet contains paracetamol 100 mg[a,b]

		Age		
0–6 months	7–11 months	12–23 months	2–4 years	5–9 years

WHO 95642

[a] For example, if your patient is aged between 2 and 4 years, you should give 2 tablets.

[b] The dose may be repeated every 4 hours until the body temperature is normal. Do not give more than four doses on the same day.

Table 5
How many paracetamol tablets you should give if each tablet contains paracetamol 500 mg[a,b]

Age (years)			
1–5	6–9	9–14	over 15

WHO 95643

[a] For example, if your patient is aged between 9 and 14 years, you should give 1 tablet.

[b] The dose may be repeated every 4 hours until the body temperature is normal. Do not give more than four doses on the same day.

Paracetamol and aspirin are used to lower temperature. They cannot cure malaria.

You can also lower the patient's temperature by fanning and by sponging down with tepid (slightly warm) water. These methods are particularly important for young children. They will help to bring down the temperature even if you do not have any aspirin or paracetamol.

If supervision is impossible

It may be impossible to supervise the whole course of treatment if the patient lives far away. In this case, it is very important to make sure the patient (or parent) knows how to take (or give) the medicine correctly:

1. Watch the patient swallow the first dose: make sure the correct number of tablets or spoonfuls is taken.
2. Check that the patient does not vomit after taking the medicine (watch for 30 minutes). (If the patient vomits, proceed as described on page 37.)
3. Give the patient the correct number of tablets or amount of syrup (to take home) for day 2 and day 3.
4. Explain that it is very important to take the full dosage for

day 2 and day 3, otherwise malaria will soon return (see below—"Underdosing").

5. Explain that it is dangerous to take all the tablets or syrup at once. The tablets and syrup should be kept out of the reach of children.

Underdosing

Some people stop taking medicine after one or two days because:

* They think it is dangerous to take medicine when they feel better—*this is not true.*
* They want to save the rest of the tablets for the next time they become sick—*if they do this, they will probably become sick again sooner than they expect!*
* The medicine may cause unwanted effects on the body—*see below*.

If the patient does not take the full treatment, there will not be enough medicine in the blood to kill all the malaria parasites. This is called *underdosing*. Underdosing can also happen if the patient vomits the medicine.

Patients who do not take the full treatment may feel better at first, but their bodies still contain a few malaria parasites. These parasites will multiply and will make the patients sick again within days or weeks. Underdosing is one of the most common reasons for treatment failure (people who come back with signs of malaria after taking treatment).

When you give standard malaria treatment, always explain to people that they *must* take the full number of tablets (or spoons of syrup) for the full 3 days, otherwise they will get malaria again soon

---

Unwanted effects of chloroquine

Some people feel itchy after taking chloroquine—you may see them scratching. You may find that a lump of sugar taken with the tablets will prevent this. Occasionally chloroquine may cause nausea, vomiting, and difficulties in seeing things clearly. These effects are not dangerous, and they will go away soon after the 3-day treatment is completed. People who have these effects must still continue the *full* treatment, otherwise they will not be cured.

What to do if standard malaria treatment fails

Suppose that a sick person comes to you for treatment. You recognize malaria and give standard malaria treatment. You watch the patient swallow the first dose and the patient goes home with tablets for day 2 and day 3. *Within 14 days* after starting treatment the patient comes back to you with features of malaria *again*.

The patient described above is an example of *treatment failure*. Some patients feel better after taking the treatment, and then become ill again within 14 days. Other patients do not improve 48 hours after starting treatment. Both types of patient are examples of treatment failure.

Action

Do the following in the order shown:

1. First, check that the patient took the full treatment. Did the patient take chloroquine on all three days? Did the patient take the dose on each day?
2. If the patient *did* take the full treatment, refer the patient to a clinic or hospital as soon as possible.
3. If the patient did *not* take the full treatment (or vomited within 30 minutes after taking the medicine—on one or several occasions), he or she has treatment failure due to underdosing. Give standard malaria treatment again. Supervise the patient for 3 days—watch the patient swallow the medicine each day until the treatment is completed. Check each day whether the patient improves. If there is no improvement (or vomiting continues), refer the patient to a clinic or hospital as soon as possible.

Severe malaria

If you think a patient has severe malaria (see pages 24–25) do the following:

1. *Give the first dose of chloroquine* (standard malaria treatment—see Tables 1, 2, and 3 on pages 31–32). If the patient is very ill, it may be difficult to swallow the tablets. It may be easier to crush the tablets and mix the powder with water, or to give chloroquine syrup. *Try very hard* to get the patient to take the medicine, but do not force it into the patient's throat if he or she cannot swallow.
2. *Bring down the fever.* Give paracetamol or aspirin (see Tables 4 and 5 on pages 33–34). Take off most of the patient's clothes and moisten the body with tepid (slightly warm) water, using a sponge or cloth. Get someone to fan the patient continuously (including during the journey to the clinic or hospital). Protect the patient from direct sunlight.
3. *Move the patient to the nearest clinic or hospital as soon as possible.* **Do not wait**, even when it is night-time. This is a matter of life or death!
4. *Write a referral note.* Write down the patient's details, what you have observed, and (most importantly) what medicines you have given—how many tablets of each medicine, and what time they were given. Give the note to the person who is taking the patient, so that the health workers at the clinic or hospital know what medicines the patient has taken.

Special groups, special care

Pregnant women

When a woman is pregnant her body is weaker and she can become ill more easily. A pregnant woman with malaria must be treated immediately, otherwise she may become very ill and may even die.

Malaria is also dangerous for the baby inside: the woman can have a miscarriage or the baby may die at birth. Even if the baby is born alive, it may be very small and weak.

Some pregnant women do not want to take chloroquine because they think it is bad for the baby inside. It is important to explain to all pregnant women that:

— **malaria is very dangerous** for the baby inside!
— **chloroquine is very safe** for a pregnant woman and it does not damage the baby inside.

If a pregnant woman has malaria, she must take the full treatment—otherwise some malaria parasites will survive in the blood, and she will get malaria again. This is very bad for the baby. **Therefore she must take the full dose of chloroquine for the full 3 days of treatment!**

Note: Prevention is better than cure. Always advise pregnant women to sleep under a mosquito net and to go to bed early each evening (see page 14).

Children

Let us look again at what is important for children:

* A child's body is weaker than an adult's body against malaria. This is why many of your patients will be children, and many of these children will be very ill.
* Very sick children must always be sent to a clinic or hospital,

but you should always start treatment yourself if you think a child has malaria (see "Severe malaria", page 38).

- When children come to you for treatment you should always pay attention to their breathing.
- Be certain to hand out the correct amount of medicine, according to the treatment schedules.
- Always advise parents to keep medicine at home out of children's reach.
- Children under the age of 2 years may have many diseases besides malaria.
- Children with fever in high-risk areas or at high-risk times of year should be started on standard malaria treatment and then referred to the nearest clinic or hospital if there are any signs of severe malaria, or if they do not get better within 48 hours.

Recording and reporting

In some countries the community health worker must record and report all cases of malaria.

It is very important to fill in all forms promptly and completely. District health staff need this information in order to know:

— how much malaria is in your community, and when, so that they can provide you with enough medicines at the right time;
— whether your village has more malaria cases than usual for the time of year, so that necessary control measures can be carried out;
— whether treatment failures reported by you are due to malaria or to other causes.

In order to have this information available you need to fill in the *day-book* and *monthly summary report* regularly.

Day-book

The day-book is a register (form) that contains information about each patient on: the date of examination; the complaint (symptoms); the community health worker's findings; the patient's name, age, and sex; and the action taken—treatment (including dosage), response to treatment, and referral.

Monthly summary report

The monthly summary report summarizes information on the number of malaria cases seen each month. It should include information on severe cases, referred cases, treatment failures, amount of drugs used, and amount of drugs remaining for future use. If you have difficulties in filling in this report, your medical supervisor will help you.

Annex 1

How to organize your antimalaria work

Your work will be easier and more effective if you follow a few simple rules:

Rule 1

Keep your forms complete and up-to-date

- Filling in the forms will help you to make the right decisions without forgetting anything ("Should I treat this person, yes or no?" "Should I refer the person to a clinic, yes or no?").
- The forms will tell you how many people you have treated.
- If people come back with signs of malaria you can easily check the date when you gave them their last treatment and find out whether these are cases of treatment failure.
- Discussing cases with your supervisor becomes much easier if you always write down details of your cases.

Rule 2

Keep close contact with your supervisor

When you see your supervisor, do the following:

- Go through the day-book and discuss any problematic cases.
- Go through the list of contents of your treatment kit (see page 5) to see whether anything needs to be supplied.
- Discuss anything in this manual that you do not understand.
- Discuss any other problems that you have. Sometimes (despite the information in this manual) you may not be sure how to treat a particular patient—your supervisor will be glad to help you. The supervisor may also be in a better

position to discuss your work or other health problems with the village head, village health committee, and other people in your village.

> **Do not be afraid to ask questions**

Rule 3

If you leave the village for a couple of days, tell the people where they should go if they become sick (usually, this will be the nearest health worker)

Rule 4

Share your knowledge with others

- If there are people in your community who sell antimalaria drugs, try to establish a good relationship with them. Firstly, observe how they work or ask them how they recognize and treat malaria. If they do not do this correctly, try in a friendly way and *in private* to explain to them what you have learned about the disease and its treatment. Describe to them the danger signs of severe malaria, and emphasize that patients with severe malaria (especially children) require special care and treatment. Tell them about the nearest clinic or hospital where patients with severe malaria should be referred for special treatment. Also advise them to refer patients whose condition does not improve after malaria treatment.
- Explain to drug vendors that this honest approach will be good for their business and reputation because it shows that they care about people's health and know about the drugs they sell.

Annex 2
How to organize your village

Suppose that you fill in some pools of water around your house, get your house screened, make the area around the house clean, and so on. If the people next door do not do the same, you will still get malaria because mosquitos will continue to breed in the

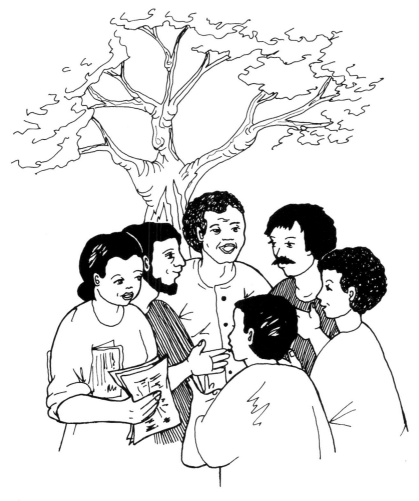

Figure 8

pools around their houses. This is why it is important that *everybody* in the village helps to improve the situation. This is true not only for malaria, but also for many other diseases carried by mosquitos.

The village must therefore be organized so that everybody works together. The village health committee can work with you to organize and lead activities to improve the health of the community and to make sure that these activities are carried out properly (Fig. 8).

During village meetings you can tell others about what you have learned as a community health worker. You can use health education materials (given to you during your training course or with the treatment kit) to explain malaria to the people and help convince them of what to do.

You or the village health committee can contact the health authorities (directly or through your supervisor) to help you organize your village and give you some ideas or advice on what can be done. You can seek help from the district council, the health inspector, the malaria specialist, the health educator, or anybody else you can think of who may be willing to help and advise you.

> **Ask the health authorities in your district to help you organize your village**